MW01232963

The Most Wanted Keto Slow Cooker Recipes

50+ Ideas For Your Healthy And Delicious Everyday Low Carb Meals

Elena Johnson

© Copyright 2021 - All rights reserved

.

The content contained within this book may not be reproduced, duplicated or transmitted without direct written permission from the author or the publisher.

Under no circumstances will any blame or legal responsibility be held against the publisher, or author, for any damages, reparation, or monetary loss due to the information contained within this book. Either directly or indirectly.

Legal Notice

This book is copyright protected. This book is only for personal use. You cannot amend, distribute, sell, use, quote or paraphrase any part, or the content within this book, without the consent of the author or publisher.

Disclaimer Notice

Please note the information contained within this document is for educational and entertainment purposes only. All effort has been executed to present accurate, up to date, and reliable, complete information. No warranties of any kind are declared or implied. Readers acknowledge that the author is not engaging in the rendering of legal, financial, medical or professional advice. The content within this book has been derived from various sources. Please consult a licensed professional before attempting any techniques outlined in this book.

By reading this document, the reader agrees that under no circumstances is the author responsible for any losses, direct or indirect, which are incurred as a result of the use of information contained within this document, including, but not limited to, errors, omissions, or inaccuracies

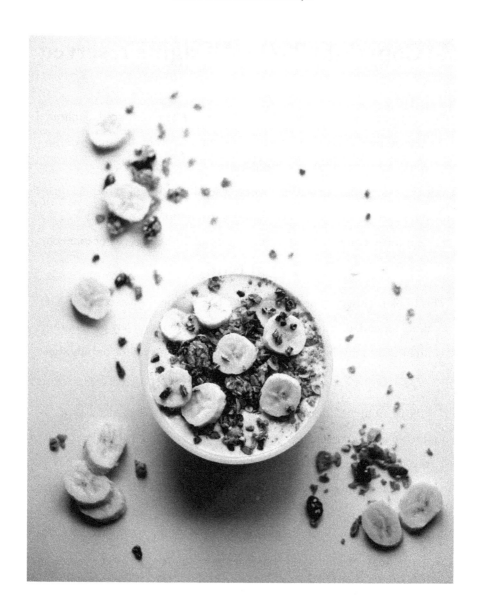

TABLE OF CONTENTS

INTRODUCTION 8

BREAKFAST 12

1. KETO SLOW COOKER TURKEY STUFFED PEPPERS 12
2. SLOW COOKER KETO 14
3. CAULIFLOWER CASSEROLE WITH TOMATO AND GOAT CHEESE 16
4. GREEK EGGS BREAKFAST CASSEROLE 18
5. SLOW COOKER TURKISH BREAKFAST EGGS 20
6. CHEESY GARLIC BRUSSELS SPROUTS 22

LUNCH 24

7. BACON WRAPPED CAULIFLOWER 24
8. CAULIFLOWER RICE 26
9. CURRY CAULIFLOWER 27
10. GARLIC CAULIFLOWER STEAKS 29
11. EGGPLANT GRATIN 30
12. MOROCCAN EGGPLANT MASH 32
13. SAUTÉED BELL PEPPERS 34
14. GARLIC ARTICHOKE 36
15. BROCCOLI STEW 37
16. SPICED FENNEL SLICES 38
17. OKRA STEW 39

DINNER 40

18. BRAISED LAMB WITH FENNEL 40
19. BEEF AND MUSHROOM GRAVY 42
20. SHORT RIBS 43
21. SWEET AND SPICY POTATO CHILI 44

22. Beef Tongue Tacos 46

23. Breakfast Casserole 48

24. Birria De Res 50

25. Vegetable Beef 52

26. Meatballs 54

27. Beef Chili 56

28. Chuck Roast 58

29. Beef Steak With Peppers 60

MEAT RECIPES 62

30. Chili Lime Beef 62

POULTRY 64

31. Chicken Curry 64

SIDE DISH RECIPES 66

32. Lemon Artichokes 66

33. Mashed Potatoes 67

VEGETABLES 68

34. Familiar Mediterranean Dish 68

35. Artichoke Pasta 70

36. Veggie Lasagna 72

37. Aloo Gobi 74

38. Jackfruit Carnitas 76

39. Butternut Macaroni Squash 78

40. Veggie Pot Pie 80

FISH & SEAFOOD 82

41. Salmon And Radish Soup 82

APPETIZERS & SNACKS..**84**

42. CHEESE CHIPS AND GUACAMOLE 84

43. CAULIFLOWER "POTATO" SALAD 86

44. LOADED CAULIFLOWER MASHED "POTATOES" 88

45. KETO BREAD 90

DESSERT **92**

46. COCONUT, CHOCOLATE, AND ALMOND TRUFFLE BAKE 92

47. PEANUT BUTTER, CHOCOLATE AND PECAN CUPCAKES........... 94

48. VANILLA AND STRAWBERRY CHEESECAKE 96

49. COFFEE CREAMS WITH TOASTED SEED CRUMBLE TOPPING 98

50. LEMON CHEESECAKE 100

30 DAY MEAL PLAN..**102**

CONVERSION TABLES..**106**

CONCLUSION **110**

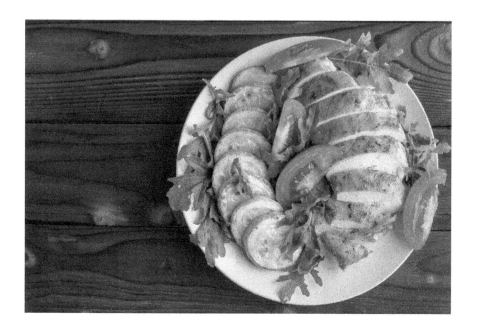

INTRODUCTION

The ketogenic diet is trendy, and for an excellent reason. It truly teaches healthy eating without forcing anyone into at risk. The success rate of keto is relatively high. While there are no specific numbers to suggest the exact rate, it is only fair to state that those who have the will to change their lifestyle and are okay adjusting to new eating habits, almost every one of them will make it through as a success story.

A diet that results in the production of ketone bodies by the liver is called a ketogenic diet; it causes your system to use fat instead of carbohydrates for energy. Limit your carbohydrate intake to a low level, causing some reactions. However, it is not a high protein diet. It involves moderate protein, low carbohydrate intake, and high fat intake.

Regardless of your lifestyle, everyone benefits from the keto diet in the following ways:

Weight Loss

Far more important than the visual aspect of excess weight is its negative influence on your body. Too much weight affects the efficiency of your body's blood flow, which in turn also affects how much oxygen your heart is able to pump to every part of your system. Too much weight also means that there are layers of fat covering your internal organs, which prevents them from working efficiently. It makes it hard to walk because it puts great pressure on your joints, and makes it very difficult to complete even regular daily tasks. A healthy weight allows your body to move freely and your entire internal system to work at its optimal levels.

Cognitive Focus

In order for your brain to function at its best, it needs to have balanced levels of all nutrients and molecules, because a balance allows it to focus on other things, such as working, studying, or creativity. If you eat carbs, the sudden insulin spike that comes with them will force your brain to stop whatever it was doing and to turn its focus on the correct breakdown of glucose molecules. This is why people often feel sleepy and with a foggy mind after high-carb meals. The keto diet keeps the balance strong, so that your brain does not have to deal with any sudden surprises.

Blood Sugar Control

If you already have diabetes, or are prone to it, then controlling your blood sugar is obviously of the utmost importance. However, even if you are not battling a type of diabetes at the moment, that doesn't mean that you are not in danger of developing it in the future. Most people forget that insulin is a finite resource in your body. You are given a certain amount of it, and it is gradually used up throughout your life. The more often you eat carbs, the more often your body needs to use insulin to break down the glucose; and when it reaches critically low levels of this finite resource, diabetes is formed.

Lower Cholesterol and Blood Pressure

Cholesterol and triglyceride levels maintain, or ruin, your arterial health. If your arteries are clogged up with cholesterol, they cannot efficiently transfer blood through your system, which in some cases even results in heart attacks. The keto diet keeps all of these levels at an optimal level, so that they do not interfere with your body's normal functioning.

Slow Cookers

Slow cookers are not new appliances in the culinary world. They have been around for decades; you might even have fond memories from your childhood of your parents serving your favorite dinner out of one. Slow cookers are very versatile because the cooking environment works the same no matter the cuisine. Knowing what slow cookers can and can't do is important for planning your meals, especially for a diet like keto.

Some of the reasons to use a slow cooker include:

Enhances flavor: Cooking ingredients over several hours with spices, herbs, and other seasonings creates vegetables and proteins that burst with delicious flavors. This slow process allows the flavors to mellow and deepen for an enhanced eating experience.

Saves time: Cooking at home takes a great deal of time: prepping, sautéing, stirring, turning the heat up and down, and watching the meal so that it does not over- or undercook. If you're unable to invest the time, you might find yourself reaching for convenience foods instead of healthy choices. Slow cookers allow you to do other activities while the meal cooks. You can put your ingredients in the slow cooker in the morning and come home to a perfectly cooked meal.

Convenient: Besides the time-saving aspect, using a slow cooker can free up the stove and oven for other dishes. This can be very convenient for large holiday meals or when you want to serve a side dish and entrée as well as a delectable dessert. Clean up is simple when you use the slow cooker for messy meals because most inserts are nonstick or are easily cleaned with a little soapy water, and each meal is prepared in either just the machine or using one additional vessel to sauté ingredients. There is no wide assortment of pots, pans, and baking dishes to contend with at the end of the day.

Low heat production: If you have ever cooked dinner on a scorching summer afternoon, you will appreciate the low amount of heat produced by a slow cooker. Even after eight hours of operation, slow cookers do not heat up your kitchen and you will not be sweating over the hot stovetop. Slow cookers use about a third of the energy of conventional cooking methods, just a little more energy than a traditional light bulb.

Supports healthy eating: Cooking your food at high heat can reduce the nutrition profile of your foods, breaking down and removing the majority of vitamins, minerals, and antioxidants while producing unhealthy chemical compounds that can contribute to disease. Low-heat cooking retains all the goodness that you want for your diet.

Saves Money: Slow cookers save you money because of the low amount of electricity they use and because the best ingredients for slow cooking are the less expensive cuts of beef and heartier inexpensive vegetables. Tougher cuts of meat—brisket, chuck, shanks—break down beautifully to fork-tender goodness. Another cost-saving benefit is that most 6-quart slow cookers will produce enough of a recipe to stretch your meals over at least two days. Leftovers are one of the best methods for saving money.

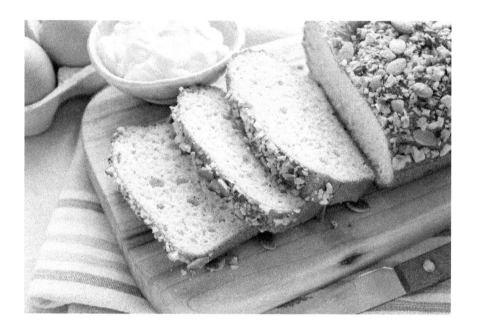

BREAKFAST

1. Keto Slow cooker Turkey Stuffed Peppers

Preparation time: 15 minutes

Cooking time: 6 hours

Servings: 7

Ingredients:

- olive oil1 tablespoon

- Ground turkey1 lb..

- onion1 pcs - garlic1 clove

- green bell peppers4 pcs

- tomato sauce/pasta sauce (low carb)24 oz.. jar

- water1/2 cup

Directions:

1. Peel and cut the small onion, peel the garlic, and press or mince it.

2. Wash the bell peppers, cut off the tops and clean them accurately.

3. Take a medium bowl, put their ground turkey, cut onion, pressed or minced garlic, and add pasta sauce.

4. Separate the compound into four equal parts, place the mixtures into the prepared cleaned peppers.

5. Spread the olive oil over the slow cooker bottom, and sides put the peppers inside, and top them with sauce.

6. Add a little water into the slow cooker, cook on low for 6-7 hours.

7. Serve with remaining sauce and enjoy.

Nutrition: Calories: 187 Carbohydrate: 1.9 g Protein: 48 g Fat: 21 g Sugar: 3gSodium: 99 mg Fiber: 13g

2. <u>Slow cooker Keto</u>

Preparation time: 15 minutes

Cooking time: 2 hours

Servings: 6

Ingredients:

- almond flour3 tablespoons

- coconut flour 1/2 tablespoon

- butter 1 tablespoon - egg 1 large

- sea salt1 pinch

- baking soda1/2 teaspoons

- salt

Directions:

1. Take a medium-sized skillet, melt the butter. It usually takes 20-30 seconds.

2. Pour coconut and almond flour, egg, salt into the melted butter and stir everything well.

3. Remove skillet from the heat and add baking soda.

4. Coat the slow cooker with cooking spray. Pour the mixture. Put on low for 2 hours. Check the readiness with a fork.

5. Remove the baked muffin from the slow cooker and eat with bacon slices, cheese, or other breakfast staples.

Nutrition: Calories: 321 Carbohydrate:5 g Protein: 23 g Fat: 13.9 g Sugar: 2.4 g Sodium: 67 mg Fiber: 11

3. Cauliflower Casserole with Tomato and Goat Cheese

Preparation time: 15 minutes

Cooking time: 3 hours

Servings: 12

Ingredients:

- cauliflower florets 6 cups

- olive oil 4 teaspoons

- dried oregano 1 teaspoon

- salt 1/2 teaspoon

- ground pepper 1/2 teaspoons

- Goat cheese crumbled 2 oz..

- The Sauce:

- olive oil 1 teaspoon

- garlic 3 cloves

- crushed tomatoes 1 (28 oz..) can

- bay leaves 2 pcs

- salt 1/4 teaspoon

- minced flat-leaf parsley 1/4 cup

Directions:

1. Grease the slow cooker with cooking spray, put the cauliflower on its bottom, and add olive oil, oregano, and pepper. Salt if desired.

2. Cook on the low setting within 2 hours until the cauliflower florets get tender and a little bit brown color.

3. For making the sauce: Take a medium-sized skillet, heat the olive oil, add garlic and cook 1 minute, stir it thoroughly all the time.

4. Add the crushed tomatoes and bay leaves; let it simmer for some minutes. Remove the bay leaves, dress with pepper and salt.

5. Put the sauce over the cauliflower florets in the slow cooker once the time is over.

6. Spread the Goat cheese over the dish, cover the slow cooker, and continue cooking for 1 hour on low. Serve warm!

Nutrition: Calories: 328 Carbohydrate: 3.5 g Protein: 23 g Fat: 11 g Sugar: 5 g Sodium: 100 mg Fiber: 13g

4. <u>**Greek Eggs Breakfast Casserole**</u>

Preparation time: 15 minutes

Cooking time: 6 hours

Servings: 9

Ingredients:

- eggs (whisked) 12 pcs

- milk 1/2 cup

- salt 1/2 teaspoon

- black pepper 1 teaspoon

- Red Onion 1 tablespoon

- Garlic 1 teaspoon

- Sun-dried tomatoes 1/2 cup

- spinach 2 cups

- Feta Cheese 1/2 cup crushed

- pepper at will

Directions:

1. Whisk the eggs in a bowl.

2. Add to the mixture milk, pepper, salt, and stir to combine. Add the minced onion and garlic.

3. Add dried tomatoes and spinach. Pour all the batter into the slow cooker, add Feta cheese. Set to cook on the low setting within 5-6 hours. Serve.

Nutrition: Calories: 365 Carbohydrate: 1.9 g Protein: 23 g Fat: 34 g Sugar: 3.4 g Sodium: 32 mg Fiber: 11

5. <u>Slow cooker Turkish Breakfast Eggs</u>

Preparation time: 15 minutes

Cooking time: 4 hours

Servings: 9

Ingredients:

- olive oil 1 tablespoon

- onions 2 pcs, chopped

- red bell pepper 1 pcs, sliced

- red chili 1 small - cherry tomatoes 8 pcs

- keto bread 1 slice

- eggs 4 pcs - milk 2 tablespoons

- small bunch of parsley, chopped

- natural yogurt 4 tablespoon

- pepper at will

Directions:

1. Grease the slow cooker using oil.

2. Heat-up, the oil, add the onions, pepper, and chili in a large skillet, then stir. Cook until the veggies begin to soften.

3. Transfer it in the Slow Cooker, then add the cherry tomatoes and bread, stir everything well.

4. Cook on low for 4 hours—season with fresh parsley and yogurt.

Nutrition: Calories: 123 Carbohydrate: 3.5 g Protein: 32 g Fat: 19 g Sugar: 3.4 g Sodium: 100 mg Fiber: 13g

6. <u>Cheesy Garlic Brussels Sprouts</u>

Preparation time: 15 minutes

Cooking time: 3 hours

Servings: 6

Ingredients:

- 1tablespoon unsalted butter

- 21/2 pounds Brussels sprouts, trimmed and halved

- 3/4 cup grated Parmesan cheese

- 2tablespoons heavy cream

- 1/8teaspoon freshly grated nutmeg

- 4cloves garlic, thinly sliced

- 4ounces cream cheese, cubed

- 1/2teaspoon kosher salt

- 1/4teaspoon ground black pepper

Directions:

1. Coat the insert of a 4- to – 6-quart slow cooker with the butter. Add the garlic, cream cheese, Brussels sprouts, pepper, and salt.

2. Toss to mix very well—cover and cook on the low, about 2 to 3 hours.

3. Turn off the slow cooker. Stir in cream, parmesan, and nutmeg until the cheeses thaw and the Brussels sprouts are coated in a creamy sauce. Taste, season with more pepper if required. Serve.

Nutrition: Calories: 356 Carbohydrate: 1.0 g Protein: 23 g Fat: 34 g Sugar: 3.4 g Sodium: 56 mg Fiber: 9

LUNCH

7. Bacon Wrapped Cauliflower

Preparation time: 15 minutes

Cooking time: 7 hours

Servings: 4

Ingredients:

- 11 oz. cauliflower head

- 3 oz. bacon, sliced

- 1 teaspoon salt

- 1 teaspoon cayenne pepper

- 1 oz. butter, softened

- 3/4 cup water

Directions:

1. Sprinkle the cauliflower head with the salt and cayenne pepper then rub with butter.

2. Wrap the cauliflower head in the sliced bacon and secure with toothpicks.

3. Pour water in the slow cooker and add the wrapped cauliflower head.

4. Cook the cauliflower head for 7 hours on Low.

5. Then let the cooked cauliflower head cool for 10 minutes.

6. Serve it!

Nutrition: Calories 187, Fat 14.8, Fiber 2.1, Carbs 4.7, Protein 9.5

8. <u>Cauliflower Rice</u>

Preparation time: 15 minutes

Cooking time: 2 hours

Servings: 5

Ingredients:

- 1-pound cauliflower

- 1 teaspoon salt

- 1 tablespoon turmeric

- 1 tablespoon butter

- 3/4 cup water

Directions:

1. Chop the cauliflower into tiny pieces to make cauliflower rice. You can also pulse in a food processor to get very fine grains of 'rice'.

2. Place the cauliflower rice in the slow cooker.

3. Add salt, turmeric, and water.

4. Stir gently and close the lid.

5. Cook the cauliflower rice for 2 hours on High.

6. Strain the cauliflower rice and transfer it to a bowl.

7. Add butter and stir gently.

8. Serve it!

Nutrition: Calories 48, Fat 2.5, Fiber 2.6, Carbs 5 g Protein 1.9

9. <u>Curry Cauliflower</u>

Preparation time: 15 minutes

Cooking time: 5 hours

Servings: 2

Ingredients:

- 10 oz. cauliflower

- 1 teaspoon curry paste

- 1 teaspoon curry powder

- 1/2 teaspoon dried cilantro

- 1 oz. butter

- 3/4 cup water

- 1/4 cup chicken stock

Directions:

1. Chop the cauliflower roughly and sprinkle it with the curry powder and dried cilantro.

2. Place the chopped cauliflower in the slow cooker.

3. Mix the curry paste with the water.

4. Add chicken stock and transfer the liquid to the slow cooker.

5. Add butter and close the lid.

6. Cook the cauliflower for 5 hours on Low.

7. Strain 1/2 of the liquid off and discard. Transfer the cauliflower to serving bowls.

8. Serve it!

Nutrition: Calories 158, Fat 13.3, Fiber 3.9, Carbs 1.9, Protein 3.3

10. Garlic Cauliflower Steaks

Preparation time: 15 minutes

Cooking time: 3 hours

Servings: 4

Ingredients:

- 14 oz. cauliflower head
- 1 teaspoon minced garlic
- 4 tablespoons butter
- 4 tablespoons water
- 1 teaspoon paprika

Directions:

1. Wash the cauliflower head carefully and slice it into the medium steaks.
2. Mix up together the butter, minced garlic, and paprika.
3. Rub the cauliflower steaks with the butter mixture.
4. Pour the water in the slow cooker.
5. Add the cauliflower steaks and close the lid.
6. Cook the vegetables for 3 hours on High.
7. Transfer the cooked cauliflower steaks to a platter and serve them immediately!

Nutrition: Calories 129, Fat 11.7, Fiber 2.7, Carbs 5, Protein 2.2

11. <u>Eggplant Gratin</u>

Preparation time: 15 minutes

Cooking time: 5 hours

Servings: 7

Ingredients:

- 1 tablespoon butter
- 1 teaspoon minced garlic
- 2 eggplants, chopped
- 1 teaspoon salt
- 1 tablespoon dried parsley
- 4 oz. Parmesan, grated
- 4 tablespoons water
- 1 teaspoon chili flakes

Directions:

1. Mix the dried parsley, chili flakes, and salt together.
2. Sprinkle the chopped eggplants with the spice mixture and stir well.
3. Place the eggplants in the slow cooker.
4. Add the water and minced garlic.
5. Add the butter and sprinkle with the grated Parmesan.
6. Close the lid and cook the gratin for 5 hours on Low.

7. Open the lid and cool the gratin for 10 minutes.

8. Serve it.

Nutrition: Calories 107, Fat 5.4, Fiber 5.6, Carbs 1.0, Protein 6.8

12. Moroccan Eggplant Mash

Preparation time: 15 minutes

Cooking time: 7 hours

Servings: 4

Ingredients:

- 1 eggplant, peeled

- 1 jalapeno pepper

- 1 teaspoon curry powder

- 1/2 teaspoon salt

- 1 teaspoon paprika

- 3/4 teaspoon ground nutmeg

- 2 tablespoons butter

- 3/4 cup almond milk

- 1 teaspoon dried dill

Directions:

1. Chop the eggplant into small pieces.

2. Place the eggplant in the slow cooker.

3. Chop the jalapeno pepper and combine it with the eggplant.

4. Then sprinkle the vegetables with the curry powder, salt, paprika, ground nutmeg, and dried dill.

5.   Add almond milk and butter.

6.   Close the lid and cook the vegetables for 7 hours on Low.

7.   Cool the vegetables and then blend them until smooth with a hand blender.

8.   Transfer the cooked eggplant mash into the bowls and serve!

Nutrition: Calories 190, Fat 17, Fiber 5.6, Carbs 1.0, Protein 2.5

13. Sautéed Bell Peppers

Preparation time: 15 minutes

Cooking time: 5 hours

Servings: 6

Ingredients:

- 8 oz. bell peppers

- 7 oz. cauliflower, chopped

- 2 oz. bacon, chopped

- 1 teaspoon salt

- 1 teaspoon ground black pepper

- 3/4 cup coconut milk, unsweetened

- 1 teaspoon butter

- 1 teaspoon thyme

- 1 onion, diced

- 1 teaspoon turmeric

Directions:

1. Remove the seeds from the bell peppers and chop them roughly.

2. Place the bell peppers, cauliflower, and bacon in the slow cooker.

3. Add the salt, ground black pepper, coconut milk, butter, milk, and thyme.

4. Stir well then add the diced onion.

5. Add the turmeric and stir the mixture.

6. Close the lid and cook 5 hours on Low.

7. When the meal is cooked, let it chill for 10 minutes and serve it!

Nutrition: Calories 195, Fat 12.2, Fiber 4.2, Carbs 3.1, Protein 6.7

14. Garlic Artichoke

Preparation time: 15 minutes

Cooking time: 2 hours

Servings: 4

Ingredients:

- 8 oz. artichoke, trimmed, chopped

- 2 teaspoons butter

- 1 garlic clove, peeled

- 1/4 cup water

- 1/2 teaspoon ground black pepper

Directions:

1. Chop the garlic clove.

2. Melt the butter and mix it with the chopped garlic.

3. Add the ground black pepper and stir the mixture.

4. Place the artichoke in the slow cooker and cover it with the butter mixture.

5. Add water and close the lid.

6. Cook the artichoke for 2 hours on High.

7. Transfer the cooked artichoke to a platter and serve!

Nutrition: Calories 45, Fat 2, Fiber 3.2, Carbs 4.6, Protein 2

15. Broccoli Stew

Preparation time: 15 minutes

Cooking time: 6 hours

Servings: 3

Ingredients:

- 6 oz. broccoli, chopped

- 1 cup spinach

- 3/4 cup almond milk, unsweetened

- 2 oz. white cabbage, shredded

- 1 tablespoon butter

- 1 teaspoon salt

- 1 teaspoon white pepper

- 2 cups water

Directions:

1. Chop the spinach and place it in the slow cooker.

2. Add chopped broccoli, almond milk, shredded cabbage, butter, salt, water and white pepper. Stir the ingredients and close the lid.

3. Cook the stew for 6 hours on Low.

4. Stir the stew gently and transfer to serving bowls.

Nutrition: Calories 200, Fat 18.4, Fiber 3.7, Carbs 5, Protein 3.6

16. Spiced Fennel Slices

Preparation time: 15 minutes

Cooking time: 2 hours

Servings: 5

Ingredients:

- 1-pound fennel bulb.

- 1 teaspoon cumin

- 1 teaspoon thyme

- 1 teaspoon salt

- 1 oz. butter

- 1 tablespoon olive oil

Directions:

1. Mix the cumin, thyme, salt, and olive oil.

2. Slice the fennel bulb. and sprinkle it with the spice mixture.

3. Place the fennel in the slow cooker and add butter.

4. Close the lid and cook for 2 hours on High.

5. Serve the meal hot!

Nutrition: Calories 95, Fat 7.7, Fiber 2.9, Carbs 3.9, Protein 1.

17. Okra Stew

Preparation time: 15 minutes

Cooking time: 5 hours

Servings: 4

Ingredients:

- 10 oz. okra, chopped

- 1 onion, diced

- 5 oz. cauliflower, chopped

- 1 cup water

- 1 teaspoon butter

- 1 teaspoon paprika

- 1/2 teaspoon ground black pepper

- 1 teaspoon dried dill

Directions:

1. Mix the chopped okra, diced onion, cauliflower, and spices.

2. Stir the mixture and place it in the slow cooker.

3. Add water and butter and close the lid.

4. Cook the stew for 5 hours on Low.

5. Transfer the dish into serving bowls and serve!

Nutrition: Calories 59, Fat 1.3, Fiber 4.1, Carbs 0.3, Protein 2.5

DINNER

18. Braised Lamb with Fennel

Preparation Time: 10 minutes

Cooking time: 7 hour.

Servings: 6

Ingredients

- 11/2 pounds lamb stew meat, cut into 2-inch pieces

- 1teaspoon kosher salt

- 1/2 teaspoon freshly ground black pepper

- 1/4 cup (1/2 stick) unsalted butter, Ghee (here), or coconut oil

- 1 onion, sliced

- 1 cup sliced fennel

- 1 (14.5-ounce) can diced tomatoes, drained

- 1/2 cup dry red wine

- 1/2tablespoons tomato paste

- 2garlic cloves, minced

- 2 teaspoons paprika

- Pinch stevia powder

- 1 cinnamon stick

- 1 cup heavy (whipping) cream

- 3/4 cup chopped pistachios

- 2 tablespoons chopped fresh mint

Directions:

1. Season the lamb with the salt and pepper.

2. In a large skillet, heat the butter over medium-high heat. Add the lamb and cook until browned on all sides, about 8 minutes. Transfer the meat to the slow cooker.

3. Return the skillet to medium-high heat and add the onion and fennel. Sauté until softened, about 3 minutes.

4. Stir in the tomatoes, red wine, tomato paste, garlic, paprika, stevia, and cinnamon. Bring to a boil. Transfer the sauce to the cooker. Cover and cook for 8 hours on low.

5. Just before serving, discard the cinnamon stick and stir in the heavy cream. Serve hot, garnished with the pistachios and mint.

Nutrition: Calories: 165 Fat: 5 g Carbs: 1 g Protein: 11 g

19. Beef and Mushroom Gravy

Preparation Time: 10 minutes

Cooking time: 8 hour.

Servings: 8

Ingredients

- 2 medium onions, peeled, sliced

- 2 pounds boneless beef round steak, slice in 8 portions

- 3 cups sliced mushrooms

- 1 cup sliced turnips

- 1 jar beef gravy

- 1 envelope dry mushroom gravy mix

Directions

1. Lay onions along bottom of slow cooker, place slices of steak on top

2. Top with sliced turnips

3. Combine beef gravy, mushroom gravy in a bowl, stir

4. Pour in slow cooker

5. Cover with lid, and cook on SLOW 8 hours

6. Serve with mashed potatoes

Nutrition: Calories: 1336 Fat: 85g Carbohydrates: 2.1g Protein: 112g

20. Short Ribs

Preparation Time: 6 minutes

Cooking time: 3 hour.

Servings: 6

Ingredients

- 1 beef short rib

- 2 small red onion

- 2 minced garlic cloves

- 1 teaspoon ground ginger

- 2 pieces star anise

- 1 tablespoon date paste

Preparation:

1. Chop the onion and crush the garlic

2. Add the beef to your slow cooker

3. Add garlic, onion, ginger, date paste and star anise on top

4. Add 1 cup water to slow cooker

5. Cover with lid, and cook on SLOW 6 hours

6. Once done, season and serve with your veggies!

Nutrition: Calories: 105 Fat: 7g Carbohydrates: 0g Protein: 11g

21. <u>Sweet And Spicy Potato Chili</u>

Preparation Time: 10 minutes

Cooking time: 4 hour.

Servings: 6

Ingredients

- 2 pounds ground beef

- 1 minced garlic clove

- 1 diced onion

- 2 cans tomato sauce

- 1 can minced tomatoes

- 3 cups beef broth

- 2 large peeled, diced sweet potatoes

- 3-4 tablespoon chili powder

- 2 teaspoon black pepper

- 1/4 teaspoon oregano

- Cilantro for garnish

Directions

1. Heat a large skillet, brown the ground beef. Drain any excess fat

2. Transfer cooked beef to slow cooker, and add rest of listed Ingredients

3. Stir well

4. Cover with lid, and cook on SLOW 4 hours

5. Serve on a platter, garnish with cilantro

Nutrition: Calories: 123 Fat 9 g Carbohydrates: 2 g Protein: 15g

22. Beef Tongue Tacos

Preparation Time: 10 minutes

Cooking time: 8 hour.

Servings: 4

Ingredients

- 1 yellow onion, cut into large slices

- 1 x 5 pound beef tongue

- 1 teaspoon sea salt

- 1 teaspoon black pepper

- 1/2 teaspoon garlic powder

- 1/2 teaspoon chipotle chili powder

- 1/4 teaspoon white pepper

- Large lettuce leaves for wraps

- Topping

- 1 jar pico de gallo

- 1-2 cups guacamole

Directions

1. Place onion slices along bottom of slow cooker

2. Sprinkle and rub seasoning over beef tongue

3. Transfer to cooker

4. Add enough water to cover meat

5. Cover with lid, and cook on LOW 8 hours

6. Once meat is cooked, remove, pull off skin

7. Discard skin and onions

8. Shred the meat, and place in lettuce wraps

9. Top with pico de gallo and guacamole

Nutrition: Calories: 195 Fat: 4g Carbohydrates: 1.6g Protein: 15g

23. Breakfast Casserole

Preparation Time: 10 minutes

Cooking time: 4 hour.

Servings: 4

Ingredients

- 1 pound cooked, bacon, chopped

- 1 diced red onion

- 1 diced bell pepper

- 1 tablespoon coconut oil

- 2 medium sweet potatoes, grated

- 2 minced garlic cloves

- 12 eggs

- 1 cup coconut milk

- 1 teaspoon dill

- Pinch crushed red pepper

- Salt, pepper to taste

- Garnish: avocado slices

Directions

1. Grease slow cooker with ghee or coconut oil

2. Combine grated sweet potato and crushed red peppers in a bowl

3. Take a skillet, heat up ghee

4. Sauté garlic, pepper, and onions 3 minutes

5. Spread layer of grated sweet potatoes, onion mixture, bacon crumble

6. Repeat until ingredients used

7. In a bowl, whisk coconut milk, eggs, and seasoning

8. Pour mixture over layers in slow cooker

9. Cover with lid, and cook on LOW 4 hours

10. Cut in rectangles, serve hot with avocado

Nutrition: Calories: 369 Fat: 23g Carbohydrates: 1.7g Protein: 20g

24. Birria De Res

Preparation Time: 10 minutes

Cooking time: 6 hour.

Servings: 8

Ingredients

- 2 pounds extra lean top round beef roast

- 3 dried guajillo peppers

- 2 dried pasilla chilies

- 2 dried ancho chilies

- 1 teaspoon cumin

- 1/4 teaspoon pepper

- 3 minced garlic cloves

- 1/2 teaspoon salt

- 11/2 cups chicken broth

- 4 chopped tomatoes

Directions

1. Take a heavy saucepan and place it over medium heat

2. Add dried chilies and stir fry 3-4 minutes until fragrant

3. Add chicken broth to saucepan

4. Cover, turn off the heat, let it sit 30 minutes

5. Seed and devein the chilies

6. Add chilies, tomatoes, water, garlic, cumin, salt, pepper to a blender, blend until smooth

7. Place roast in slow cooker, pour sauce over meat

8. Cover with lid, cook on LOW 8 hours

9. Shred with forks once cooked

Nutrition: Calories: 198 Fat: 12g Carbohydrates: 5g Protein: 28g

25. <u>Vegetable Beef</u>

Preparation Time: 8 minutes

Cooking time: 6 hour.

Servings: 20

Ingredients

- 3-4 pounds beef roast

- 1/2 teaspoon salt

- 1/4 teaspoon pepper

- Flavorless cooking oil

- 11/2 pounds red potatoes

- 1 small white onion

- 11/2 pounds carrots, peeled, cut

- 1 minced garlic clove

- 1 teaspoon dried thyme

- 1 teaspoon dried oregano

- 1/3 cup balsamic vinegar

Directions

1. Sprinkle seasoning, salt, pepper over the roast

2. Place a pan over medium high heat, heat the oil

3. Brown roast on all sides

4. Transfer roast to slow cooker

5. Add diced onion and potatoes around roast

6. Drizzle balsamic and vinegar over roast, add the carrots on top

7. Cover with lid, and cook on LOW 8 hours

8. Once cooked, shred the meat, and serve with potatoes, carrots, onions

9. Drizzle cook juice over top

Nutrition: Calories: 300 Fat: 8g Carbohydrates: 2.6g Protein: 24g

26. Meatballs

Preparation Time: 10 minutes

Cooking time: 7 hour.

Servings: 6

Ingredients

- 11/4 pound lean ground beef (85% lean)

- 1 egg

- 1/4 cup blanched almond flour

- 3/4 teaspoon sea salt

- 2 teaspoon onion powder

- 1/2 teaspoon garlic powder

- 1 tablespoon Italian seasoning blend

- Pinch crushed red pepper

- 1 tablespoon chopped fresh parsley

- Marinara

- 1 can (28 oz.) crushed tomatoes with basil

- 1 can (14 oz.) diced tomatoes with basil and garlic

- 1 can (6 ounce) tomato paste

- 2 cloves fresh garlic, chopped

- 2 tablespoons chopped fresh oregano leaves

- 2 bay leaves

- Pinch of sea salt, pepper

Directions

1. Take a small bowl and add almond flour, onion, 1/2 a teaspoon salt, onion, Italian seasoning, red pepper, garlic powder, mix well

2. Take a large bowl and add ground beef

3. Add the egg and almond mixture to the beef, and mix well

4. Using your hand, form 2o meatballs from mixture

5. Take a large baking sheet and line with parchment paper, pre-heat broiler on oven

6. Broil meatballs 2-4 minutes per side

7. Add the sauce ingredients to slow cooker

8. Add broiled meatballs to cooker, stir

9. Cover with lid, and cook over LOW 4 hours

10. Serve with garnish of fresh herbs

Nutrition: Calories: 354 Fat: 17g Carbohydrates: 1.6g Protein: 22g

27. Beef Chili

Preparation Time: 10 minutes

Cooking time: 7 hour.

Servings: 6

Ingredients

- 1 tablespoon avocado oil

- 1 pound grass fed beef

- 1 diced green bell pepper

- 1 diced red bell pepper

- 1 large diced onion

- 2 garlic cloves, chopped

- 1 small sweet potato, peeled, diced

- 1 can (28 oz.) crushed tomatoes

- 1 can (14 oz.) diced tomatoes (fire roasted)

- 3 tablespoons chili powder

- 1 tablespoon smoked paprika, 1 tablespoon ground cumin

- 2 teaspoon salt

- 1/2 teaspoon ground cinnamon,1/2 teaspoon ground chipotle chili

- Garnish: sliced avocado, fresh cilantro

Directions

1. Take a large skillet, heat on medium

2. Heat up oil, add beef and cook 4-6 minutes, break apart as cooking

3. Transfer beef to slow cooker, stir in onion, pepper, potatoes, diced tomatoes, chili powder, smoked paprika, salt, cumin, chipotle, cinnamon

4. Cover with the lid, and cook on HIGH 6 hours

5. Serve with avocado or cilantro

Nutrition Values (Per Serving): Calories: 173 Fat: 5g Carbohydrates: 1.5g Protein: 5g

28. Chuck Roast

Preparation Time: 10 minutes

Cooking time: 7 hour.

Servings: 6

Ingredients

- 1/3 cup olive oil

- 3-4 pounds chuck roast

- 6 carrots, diced

- 3 celery stalks, diced

- 1 large onion, diced

- 4 garlic cloves, minced

- 2 peeled, cubed rutabagas

- 1 cup dried mushrooms

- 1 cup beef broth

- 1/2 cup fresh basil, 1/2 cup fresh parsley

- 1/4 cup fresh rosemary

- 2 tablespoons balsamic vinegar

- Zest from 1 lemon

- 1/3 cup pine nuts

- Pinch kosher salt, black pepper

Directions

1. Soak dried mushrooms in 1 cup lukewarm water 30 minutes

2. Strain the mushrooms, retain the liquid

3. Pour liquid through a cheesecloth, set aside

4. Heat a large skillet, add pine nuts, stir fry them 10 minutes

5. Transfer pine nuts, fresh herbs, lemon zest, garlic to food processor, pulse well

6. Drizzle in olive oil, pulse until a paste forms

7. Season the roast generously with paste, and salt and pepper

8. In same skillet, heat olive oil over high, sear roast on all sides, transfer to slow cooker

9. Pour broth into the skillet, deglaze skillet, pour liquid over roast

10. Add mushroom liquid, mushrooms, balsamic vinegar, leftover pine nut to cooker

11. Scatter carrots, onion, celery, rutabaga around the roast

12. Cover with lid, and cook on SLOW 8 hours

13. Remove roast and veggies, drizzle cooking juice over ingredients

Nutrition: Calories: 270 Fat: 21g Carbohydrates: 5g Protein: 11g

29. Beef Steak With Peppers

Preparation Time: 10 minutes

Cooking time: 7 hour.

Servings: 6

Ingredients

- 8 pieces cubed steak

- 13/4 teaspoon garlic salt

- Pinch of black pepper

- 1 can (8 oz.) tomato sauce

- 1 cup water

- 1 red bell pepper, sliced 1/4 inch strips

- 1 medium onion, sliced 1/4 inch strips

- 1/3 cup green pitted olives + 2 tablespoons brine

Directions

1. Season the beef with garlic salt, pepper

2. Transfer to slow cooker, add onion, red pepper, tomato sauce, olives

3. Pour in 2 cups water

4. Cover with lid, cook on LOW 8 hours

5. Serve over rice

Nutrition: Calories: 240 Fat: 12g Carbohydrates: 2.4g Protein: 10g

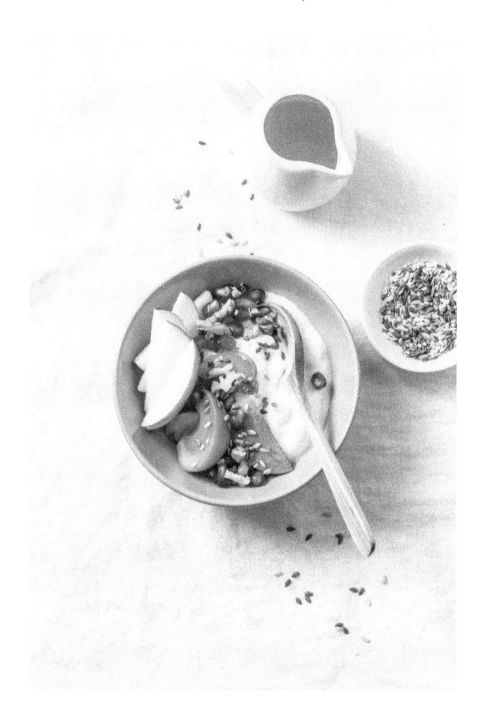

MEAT RECIPES

30. Chili Lime Beef

Preparation Time: 10 minutes

Cooking Time: 6 hours

Servings: 4

Ingredients:

- 1 lb. beef chuck roast

- 1 tsp chili powder

- 2 cups lemon-lime soda

- 1 fresh lime juice

- 1 garlic clove, crushed

- 1/2 tsp salt

Directions:

1. Place beef chuck roast into the slow cooker.

2. Season roast with garlic, chili powder, and salt.

3. Pour lemon-lime soda over the roast.

4. Cover slow cooker with lid and cook on low for 6 hours. Shred the meat using a fork.

5. Add lime juice over shredded roast and serve.

Nutrition: Calories 355 Fat 16.8 g Carbohydrates 14 g Sugar 11.3 g Protein 35.5 g Cholesterol 120 mg

POULTRY

31. Chicken Curry

Preparation Time: 10 minutes

Cooking Time: 6 hours

Servings: 6

Ingredients:

- 3 lb. chicken drumsticks and thighs
- 1 yellow onion, diced
- 2 tablespoons of butter, melted
- 1/2 cup of chicken stock
- 15 oz. canned tomatoes, crushed
- 1/4 cup of lemon juice
- 4 garlic cloves, minced
- 1 lb. spinach, chopped
- 1/2 cup of heavy cream
- 1 tablespoon of ginger, grated
- 1/2 cup of cilantro, diced
- 1 ½ teaspoon of paprika

- 1 tablespoon of cumin, ground

- 1 ½ teaspoon of coriander, ground

- 1 teaspoon of turmeric, ground

- Salt and black pepper- to taste

- A pinch cayenne peppers

Directions:

1 Start by throwing all the ingredients into the Slow cooker except lemon juice, cream, and cilantro, then mixes them well.

2 Cover it and cook for 6 hours on Low Settings.

3 Stir in remaining ingredients and cook again for 1 hour on low heat.

4 Garnish as desired.

5 Serve warm.

Nutrition: Calories 537 Total Fat 19.8 g Saturated Fat 1.4 g Cholesterol 10 mg Total Carbs 5.1 g Fiber 0.9 g Sugar 1.4 g Sodium 719 mg Potassium 374 mg Protein 37.6.8 g

SIDE DISH RECIPES

32. Lemon Artichokes

Preparation time: 15 minutes

Cooking time: 3 Hours

Servings: 2

Ingredients

- `1 cup veggie stock

- `2 medium artichokes, trimmed

- `1 tablespoon lemon juice

- `1 tablespoon lemon zest, grated

- `Salt to the taste

Directions:

1   In your Slow cooker, mix the artichokes with the stock and the other Ingredients, and then toss it, put the lid on and cook on Low for 3 hours.

2   Divide artichokes between plates and serve as a side dish.

Nutrition: calories 100, fat 2, fiber 5, carbs 10, protein 4

33. Mashed Potatoes

Preparation time: 15 minutes

Cooking time: 6 Hours

Servings: 2

Ingredients

- `1 pound gold potatoes, peeled and cubed

- `2 garlic cloves, chopped

- `1 cup milk

- `1 cup water

- `2 tablespoons butter

- `A pinch of salt and white pepper

Directions:

1 In your Slow cooker, mix the potatoes with the water, salt and pepper, put the lid on and cook on Low for 6 hours.

2 Mash the potatoes; add the rest of the Ingredients, whisk and serve.

Nutrition: calories 135, fat 4, fiber 2, carbs 10, protein 4

VEGETABLES

34. Familiar Mediterranean Dish

Preparation time: 15 minutes

Cooking time: 4 hours

Servings: 4 people

Ingredients:

- `2¼ cup unsalted vegetable broth

- `1½ cup uncooked quinoa, rinsed

- `1 (15½-oz.) can chickpeas, drained and rinsed

- `1 cup red onions, sliced

- `2 garlic cloves, minced

- `2½ tbsp. olive oil

- `Salt, to taste

- `2 tsp. fresh lemon juice

- `½ cup roasted red bell peppers, drained and chopped

- `4 cup fresh baby arugula

- `12 Kalamata olives, pitted and halved lengthwise

- `2 oz. feta cheese, crumbled

- `2 tbsp. fresh oregano, chopped

Directions:

1   In a slow cooker, place the broth, quinoa, chickpeas, onions, garlic, 1½ tsp. of the oil, and salt and stir to combine. Set the slow cooker on low and cook, covered for about 3-4 hours.

2   Meanwhile, in a bowl, add the lemon juice, remaining oil, and salt and mix well. Uncover the slow cooker and with a fork, fluff the quinoa mixture.

3   In the slow cooker, add the olive oil mixture, bell peppers, and arugula and gently combine. Over the pot for about 5 minutes before serving. Garnish with the olives, feta cheese, and oregano and serve.

Nutrition: Calories: 536 Carbohydrates: 78.5g Protein: 23.2g Fat: 16.1g

35. Artichoke Pasta

Preparation time: 15 minutes

Cooking time: 8 hours

Servings: 4 people

Ingredients:

- `3 cans diced tomatoes with basil, oregano, and garlic

- `2 cans artichoke hearts, drained and quartered

- `6 garlic cloves, minced

- `½ cup whipping cream

- `12 oz. dried fettuccine pasta

- `¼ cup pimiento-stuffed green olives

- `¼ cup feta cheese, crumbled

Directions:

1 Drain the juices from two of the cans of diced tomatoes. In a greased slow cooker, place the drained and undrained tomatoes alongside the artichoke hearts and garlic and mix well.

2 Set the slow cooker on low and cook, covered for about 6-8 hours. In a large pan of salted boiling water, cook the pasta for about 8-10 minutes or according to the package's directions.

3   Drain, then rinse under cold running water the pasta. Uncover the slow cooker and stir in the whipping cream.

4   Divide the pasta onto serving plates and top with artichoke sauce. Garnish with olives and cheese and serve.

Nutrition: Calories: 479 Carbohydrates: 82.2g Protein: 20.8g Fat: 10.4g

36. Veggie Lasagna

Preparation time: 15 minutes

Cooking time: 2 hours

Servings: 4 people

Ingredients:

- `1 package baby spinach, chopped roughly

- `3 large portobello mushroom caps, sliced thinly

- `1 small zucchini, sliced thinly

- `1 container part-skim ricotta cheese

- `1 large egg

- `1 can diced tomatoes

- `1 can of crushed tomatoes

- `3 garlic cloves, minced

- `Pinch of red pepper flakes, crushed

- `15 uncooked whole-wheat lasagna noodles

- `3 cups part-skim mozzarella, shredded and divided

Directions:

1   Put the spinach, zucchini, ricotta cheese, and egg and mix well in a large bowl. In another bowl, add both cans of tomatoes with juice, garlic, and red pepper flakes and mix well.

2   In the bottom of a generously greased slow cooker, place about 1½ cup of the tomato mixture evenly. Place 5 lasagna noodles over the tomato mixture, overlapping them slightly and breaking them to fit in the pot.

3   Put half of the ricotta batter over the noodles. Now, place about 1½ cup of the tomato mixture and sprinkle with 1 cup of the mozzarella. Repeat the layers twice.

4   Cook, covered for about 2 hours on high. Uncover the slow cooker and sprinkle with the remaining mozzarella cheese. Immediately cover the cooker for about 10 minutes before serving.

Nutrition: Calories: 289 Carbohydrates: 37.1g Protein: 18.8g Fat: 8.2g

37. Aloo Gobi

Preparation Time: 15 Minutes

Cooking Time: 5 Hours

Servings: 4

Ingredients:

- `1 large cauliflower, cut into 1-inch pieces

- `1 large russet potato, peeled and diced

- `1 medium yellow onion, peeled and diced

- `1 cup canned diced tomatoes, with juice

- `1 cup frozen peas

- `¼ cup of water

- `1 (2-inch) piece fresh ginger, peeled and finely chopped

- `1½ teaspoons minced garlic (3 cloves)

- `1 jalapeño pepper, stemmed and sliced

- `1 tablespoon cumin seeds

- `1 tablespoon garam masala

- `1 teaspoon ground turmeric

- `1 heaping tablespoon fresh cilantro

- `Cooked rice, for serving (optional)

Directions:

1   Combine the cauliflower, potato, onion, diced tomatoes, peas, water, ginger, garlic, jalapeño, cumin seeds, garam masala, and turmeric in a slow cooker; mix until well combined.

2   Cover and cook on low for 4 to 5 hours.

3   Garnish with the cilantro, and serve over cooked rice (if using).

Nutrition: Calories: 115; Total fat: <1g; Protein: 6g; Sodium: 62mg; Fiber: 6g

38. Jackfruit Carnitas

Preparation Time: 15 Minutes

Cooking Time: 8 Hours

Servings: 4

Ingredients:

- `2 (20-ounce) cans jackfruit, drained, hard pieces discarded

- `¾ cup Very Easy Vegetable Broth or store-bought

- `1 tablespoon ground cumin

- `1 tablespoon dried oregano

- `1½ teaspoons ground coriander

- `1 teaspoon minced garlic (2 cloves)

- `½ teaspoon ground cinnamon

- `2 bay leaves

- `Tortillas, for serving

- `Optional toppings: diced onions, sliced radishes, fresh cilantro, lime wedges, Nacho Cheese

Directions:

1. Combine the jackfruit, vegetable broth, cumin, oregano, coriander, garlic, cinnamon, and bay leaves in a slow cooker. Stir to combine.

2. Cover and cook on low for 8 hours or on high for 4 hours.

3   Use two forks to pull the jackfruit apart into shreds.

4   Remove the bay leaves. Serve in warmed tortillas with your favorite

taco fixings.

Nutrition: Calories: 286; Total fat: 2g; Protein: 6g; Sodium: 155mg; Fiber: 5g

39. Butternut Macaroni Squash

Preparation time: 15 minutes

Cooking time: 8 hours

Servings: 5

Ingredients:

- `1/½ cups of butternut squash, cubed

- `½ cup of chopped tomatoes

- `1/½ cups of water

- `2 cloves of minced garlic

- `A handful of fresh thyme, finely chopped

- `A handful of fresh rosemary, finely chopped

- `¼ cup of nutritional yeast

- `1 cup of non-dairy milk

- `1/½ cups of whole wheat macaroni

- `Salt and pepper

Directions:

1. Add the butternut squash, diced tomatoes, water, garlic, thyme, and rosemary to the slow cooker. Cover and cook on low within 7-9 hours.

2. Transfer the ingredients from the slow cooker into a food processor and add the nutritional yeast, half a cup of non-dairy milk, and blend.

3. Pour the ingredients back into the slow cooker, add the macaroni, cover, and cook for a further 20 minutes on high. Stir, cook for a further 25 minutes and add salt and pepper to taste. Spoon onto dishes and serve.

Nutrition: Calories: 187 Fat: 2 g Carbohydrates: 35 g Protein: 8 g

40. Veggie Pot Pie

Preparation time: 15 minutes

Cooking time: 4 hours

Servings: 6

Ingredients:

- `6 -7 cups of chopped veggies of your choice

- `½ cup of diced onions

- `4 cloves of minced garlic

- `Fresh thyme, finely chopped

- `½ cup of flour

- `2 cups of chicken broth

- `¼ cup of cornstarch

- `¼ cup of heavy cream

- `Salt and pepper

- `1 thawed frozen puff pastry sheet

- `2 tablespoons of butter

Directions:

1. Put the chopped veggies in the slow cooker, put the garlic and onions. Add the flour. Add the broth and stir until everything is well blended. Cover and cook for 3-4 hours on high.

2. In a small bowl, combine the cornstarch and ¼ cup of water and whisk thoroughly. Put the cornstarch mix in the slow cooker.

3. Add the cream, cover, and continue to cook until the mixture thickens approximately 15 minutes. Transfer the vegetable mixture into a baking dish.

4. Lay the puff pastry over the top. Melt the butter and brush it over the top of the pastry. Bake at 350 degrees for 10 minutes until the pastry turns fluffy and golden. Divide onto dishes and serve

Nutrition: Calories: 325 Fat: 0.8 g Protein: 4.5 g Carbohydrates: 6.7 g

FISH & SEAFOOD

41. Salmon and Radish Soup

Preparation Time: 10 minutes

Cooking time: 3 hours

Servings: 4

Ingredients:

- `1 cup radishes, halved
- `10 oz salmon, chopped
- `1 teaspoon lime juice
- `1 teaspoon lime zest, grated
- `½ cup of coconut milk
- `2 cups of water
- `1 teaspoon salt
- `1 teaspoon garlic, diced
- `½ teaspoon chives, chopped

Directions:

1. In the slow cooker, mix the salmon with radishes and the other ingredients.

2. Close the lid and cook the liquid for 2.5 hours on High.

3. Divide into bowls and serve.

Nutrition: calories 214, fat 5, carbs 7, protein 9

APPETIZERS & SNACKS

42. Cheese Chips And Guacamole

Preparation Time: 10 Minutes

Cooking Time: 10 minutes

Servings: 4

Ingredients:

- 1cup shredded cheese (I use Mexican blend)
- FOR THE GUACAMOLE
- 1avocado, mashed
- Juice of 1/2 lime
- 1teaspoon diced jalapeño
- 1tablespoons chopped fresh cilantro leaves
- Pink Himalayan salt
- Freshly ground black pepper

Directions:

1. Preheat the oven to 350F. Line a baking sheet with parchment paper or a silicone baking mat.

2. Add 1/4-cup mounds of shredded cheese to the pan, leaving plenty of space between them, and bake until the edges are brown and the middles have fully melted, about 7 minutes.

3. Set the pan on a cooling rack, and let the cheese chips cool for 5 minutes. The chips will be floppy when they first come out of the oven but will crisp as they cool.

4. In a medium bowl, mix together the avocado, lime juice, jalapeño, and cilantro, and season with pink Himalayan salt and pepper.

5. Top the cheese chips with the guacamole, and serve.

Nutrition: Calories: 646; Total Fat: 54g; Carbs: 1.6g;Fiber: 10gProtein: 30g

43. Cauliflower "Potato" Salad

Preparation Time: 5 Minutes

Cooking Time: 45 minutes

Servings: 4

Ingredients:

- 1/2 head cauliflower

- 1tablespoon olive oil

- Pink Himalayan salt

- Freshly ground black pepper

- 1/3 cup mayonnaise

- 1tablespoon mustard

- 1/4 cup diced dill pickles

- 1teaspoon paprika

Directions:

1. Preheat the oven to 400F. Line a baking sheet with aluminum foil or a silicone baking mat.

2. Cut the cauliflower into 1-inch pieces.

3. Put the cauliflower in a large bowl, add the olive oil, season with the pink Himalayan salt and pepper, and toss to combine.

4. Spread the cauliflower out on the prepared baking sheet and bake for 25 minutes, or just until the cauliflower begins to brown. Halfway through the cooking time, give the pan a couple of shakes or stir so all sides of the cauliflower cook.

5. In a large bowl, mix the cauliflower together with the mayonnaise, mustard, and pickles. Sprinkle the paprika on top, and chill in the refrigerator for 3 hours before serving.

Nutrition: Calories: 772; Total Fat: 74g; Carbs: 2.6g; Fiber: 10g;Protein: 10g

44. Loaded Cauliflower Mashed "Potatoes"

Preparation Time: 10 Minutes

Cooking Time: 10 minutes

Servings: 4

Ingredients:

- 1head fresh cauliflower, cut into cubes

- 2garlic cloves, minced

- 6tablespoons butter

- 1/2tablespoons sour cream

- Pink Himalayan salt

- Freshly ground black pepper

- 1cup shredded cheese (I use Colb.y Jack)

- 6bacon slices, cooked and crumbled

Directions:

1. Boil a large pot of water over high heat. Add the cauliflower. Reduce the heat to medium-low and simmer for 8 to 10 minutes, until fork-tender. (You can also steam the cauliflower if you have a steamer basket.)

2. Drain the cauliflower in a colander, and turn it out onto a paper towel–lined plate to soak up the water. Blot to remove any

remaining water from the cauliflower pieces. This step is important; you want to get out as much water as possible so the mash won't be runny.

3. Add the cauliflower to the food processor (or blender) with the garlic, butter, and sour cream, and season with pink Himalayan salt and pepper.

4. Mix for about 1 minute, stopping to scrape down the sides of the bowl every 30 seconds.

5. Divide the cauliflower mix evenly among four small serving dishes, and top each with the cheese and bacon crumbles. (The cheese should melt from the hot cauliflower. But if you want to reheat it, you can put the cauliflower in oven-safe serving dishes and pop them under the broiler for 1 minute to heat up the cauliflower and melt the cheese.)

Nutrition: Calories: 131; Total Fat: 132g; Carbs: 3.4g; Fiber: 12g; Protein: 58g

45. <u>Keto Bread</u>

Time: 5 Minutes Cooking Time: 25 minutes Servings: 4

Ingredients:

- 5tablespoons butter, at room temperature, divided

- 6large eggs, lightly beaten

- 11/2 cups almond flour

- 3teaspoons baking powder

- Pinch pink Himalayan salt

Directions:

1. Preheat the oven to 390F. Coat a 9-by-5-inch loaf pan with 1 tablespoon of butter.

2. In a large bowl, use a hand mixer to mix the eggs, almond flour, remaining 4 tablespoons of butter, baking powder, MCT oil powder (if using), and pink Himalayan salt until thoroughly blended. Pour into the prepared pan.

3. Bake for 25 minutes, or until a toothpick inserted in the center comes out clean.

4. Slice and serve.

Nutrition: Calories: 165 Total Fat: 178g; Carbs: 4.6g; Net Carbs: 27g; Fiber: 19g; Protein: 74gPer Slice Calories: 165; Total Fat: 15g; Carbs: 4g; Net Carbs: 2g; Fiber: 2g; Protein: 6g

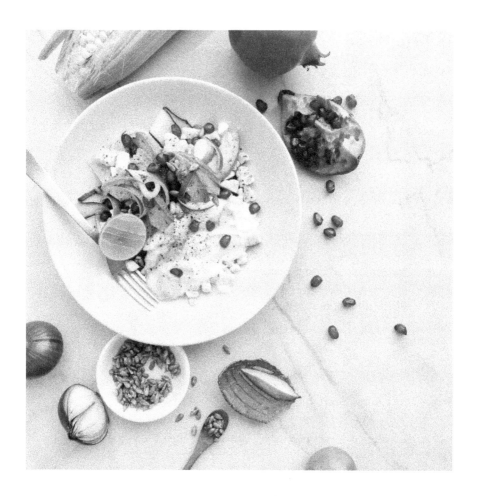

DESSERT

46. Coconut, chocolate, and almond truffle bake

Preparation Time: 10 minutes

Cooking Time: 6-8 hours

Serve: 8

Ingredients:

- `3 ounces butter, melted

- `3 ounces dark chocolate, melted

- `1 cup ground almonds

- `1 cup desiccated coconut

- `3 tbsp. unsweetened cocoa powder

- `2 tsp. vanilla extract

- `1 cup heavy cream

- `A few extra squares of dark chocolate, grated

- `1/4 cup toasted almonds, chopped

Directions:

1. In a large bowl, mix together the melted butter, chocolate, ground almonds, coconut, cocoa powder, and vanilla extract.

2. Roll the mixture into balls.

3. Grease a heat-proof dish (make sure it fits in the Slow cooker).

4. Place the balls into the dish.

5. Place the lid onto the pot and set the temperature to LOW.

6. Cook for 4 hours.

7. Leave the truffle dish to cool until warm.

8. Whip the cream until it is soft and pillowy.

9. Spread the cream over the truffle dish and sprinkle the grated chocolate and chopped toasted almonds over the top.

10. Serve immediately!

Nutrition: Calories 376, Fat 9, Carbs 1, Protein 13

47. <u>Peanut butter, chocolate and pecan cupcakes</u>

Preparation Time: 10 minutes

Cooking Time: 6-8 hours

Serve: 8

Ingredients:

- `14 paper cupcake cases

- `1 cup smooth peanut butter

- `2 ounces butter

- `2 tsp. vanilla extract

- `5 ounces dark chocolate

- `2 tbsp. coconut oil

- `2 eggs, lightly beaten

- `1 cup ground almonds

- `1 tsp. baking powder

- `1 tsp. cinnamon

- `10 pecan nuts, toasted and finely chopped

Directions:

1. Melt together the dark chocolate and coconut oil in the microwave, stir to combine and set aside.

2. Place the peanut butter and butter into a medium-sized bowl, microwave for 30 seconds at a time until the butter has just melted.

3. Stir together the peanut butter and butter until combined and smooth.

4. Stir the vanilla extract into the peanut butter mixture.

5. In a small bowl, mix together the ground almonds, eggs, baking powder, and cinnamon.

6. Pour the melted chocolate and coconut oil evenly into the 14 paper cases.

7. Spoon half of the almond/egg mixture evenly into the cases, on top of the chocolate and press down slightly.

8. Spoon the peanut butter mixture into the cases, on top of the almond/egg mixture.

9. Spoon the remaining almond/egg mixture into the cases.

10. Sprinkle the chopped pecans on top of each cupcake.

11. Very carefully place the filled cases into the Slow cooker, if they don't all fit, use a rack (so there are 2 levels of cakes).

12. Place the lid onto the pot and set the temperature to HIGH.

13. Cook for 4 hours.

14. Remove the cakes from the pot and leave to cool.

15. Serve warm, with a dollop of whipped cream!

Nutrition: Calories 14, Fat 11, Carbs 2, Protein 11

48. Vanilla and strawberry cheesecake

Preparation Time: 10 minutes

Cooking Time: 6-8 hours

Serve: 8

Ingredients:

- `Base:
- `2 ounces butter, melted
- `1 cup ground hazelnuts
- `1/2 cup desiccated coconut
- `2 tsp. vanilla extract
- `1 tsp. cinnamon
- `Filling:
- `2 cups cream cheese
- `2 eggs, lightly beaten
- `1 cup sour cream
- `2 tsp. vanilla extract
- `8 large strawberries, chopped

Directions:

1. Prepare the base: in a medium-sized bowl, combine the melted butter, hazelnuts, coconut, vanilla, and cinnamon.

2. Press the base into a greased heat-proof dish (make sure it fits into the Slow cooker).

3. In a large bowl, place the cream cheese, eggs, sour cream, and vanilla extract, beat with electric egg beaters until thick and combined.

4. Fold the strawberries through the cream cheese mixture.

5. Pour the cream cheese mixture into the dish, on top of the base, spread out until smooth.

6. Place the dish into the Slow cooker and pour enough hot water around the dish so that it comes half way up the side of the dish.

7. Place the lid onto the pot and set the temperature to LOW.

8. Cook for 6 hours until just set but slightly wobbly.

9. Allow to cool slightly before placing in the fridge until cold.

10. Serve with a dollop of whipped cream!

Nutrition: Calories 12, Fat 21, Carbs 2, Protein 11

49. Coffee creams with toasted seed crumble topping

Preparation Time: 10 minutes

Cooking Time: 6-8 hours

Serve: 8

Ingredients:

- `2 cups heavy cream

- `3 egg yolks, lightly beaten

- `1 tsp. vanilla extract

- `3 tbsp. strong espresso coffee (or 3tsp. instant coffee dissolved in 3tbsp. boiling water)

- `1/2 cup mixed seeds – sesame seeds, pumpkin seeds, chia seeds, sunflower seeds,

- `1 tsp. cinnamon

- `1 tbsp. coconut oil

Directions:

1. Heat the coconut oil in a small fry pan until melted.

2. Add the mixed seeds, cinnamon, and a pinch of salt, toss in the oil and heat until toasted and golden, place into a small bowl and set aside.

3. In a medium-sized bowl, whisk together the cream, egg yolks, vanilla, and coffee.

4. Pour the cream/coffee mixture into the ramekins.

5. Place the ramekins into the Slow cooker.

6. Pour enough hot water into the pot to reach half way up the ramekins.

7. Place the lid onto the pot and set the temperature to LOW.

8. Cook for 4 hours.

9. Remove the ramekins from the Slow cooker and leave to cool slightly on the bench.

10. Sprinkle the seed mixture over the top of each custard before serving.

Nutrition: Calories 11, Fat 12, Carbs 2, Protein 11

50. Lemon cheesecake

Preparation Time: 10 minutes

Cooking Time: 7 hours

Serve: 8

Ingredients:

- `2 ounces butter, melted
- `1 cup pecans, finely ground in the food processor
- `1 tsp. cinnamon
- `2 cups cream cheese
- `1 cup sour cream
- `2 eggs, lightly beaten
- `1 lemon
- `Few drops of stevia
- `1 cup heavy cream

Directions::

1. Mix together the melted butter, ground pecans, and cinnamon until it forms a wet, sand-like texture.

2. Press the butter/pecan mixture into a greased, heat-proof dish (make sure it fits in the Slow cooker) and set aside.

3. Place the cream cheese, eggs, sour cream, stevia, zest and juice of one lemon into a large bowl, beat with electric egg beaters until combined and smooth.

4. Pour the cream cheese mixture into the dish, on top of the base, smooth it out so that the top of the cheesecake is even.

5. Place the dish into the Slow cooker and pour enough hot water into the pot so that it reaches half way up the side of the dish.

6. Place the lid onto the pot and set the temperature to LOW.

7. Cook for 6 hours.

8. Set the cheesecake on the bench to cool and set.

9. Whip the cream until soft and pillowy, and spread over the cheesecake before serving.

Nutrition: Calories 12, Fat 9, Carbs 2, Protein 11

30 DAY MEAL PLAN

DAY	BREAKFAST	LUNCH	DINNER	DESSERTS
1	Egg Sausage Breakfast Casserole	Garlic Duck Breast	Pork Chops	Chocolate Mousse
2	Vegetable Omelet	Thyme Lamb Chops	Spicy Pork & Spinach Stew	Chocolate Chia Pudding With Almonds
3	Cheese Bacon Quiche	Autumn Pork Stew	Stuffed Taco Peppers	Coconut Macadamia Chia Pudding
4	Egg Breakfast Casserole	Handmade Sausage Stew	Chinese Pulled Pork	Keto Chocolate Mug
5	Cauliflower Breakfast Casserole	Marinated Beef Tenderloin	Bacon Wrapped Pork Loin	Vanilla Chia Pudding
6	Veggie Frittata	Chicken Liver Sauté	Lamb Barbacoa	Choco Lava Cake
7	Feta Spinach Quiche	Chicken In Bacon	Balsamic Pork Tenderloin	Coconut Cup Cakes
8	Cauliflower Mashed	Whole Chicken	Spicy Pork	Easy Chocolate Cheesecake
9	Kalua Pork With Cabbage	Duck Rolls	Zesty Garlic Pulled Pork	Chocolate Chip Brownie
10	Creamy Pork	Keto Adobo	Ranch	Coconut

	Chops	Chicken	Pork Chops	Cookies
11	Beef Taco Filling	Cayenne Pepper Drumsticks	Pork Chile Verde	Choco Pie
12	Flavorful Steak Fajitas	Keto Bbq Chicken Wings	Ham Soup	Keto Blueberry Muffins
13	Garlic Herb Pork	Sweet Corn Pilaf	Beef And Broccoli	Keto Oven-Baked Brie Cheese
14	Garlic Thyme Lamb Chops	Mediterranean Vegetable Mix	Korean Barbecue Beef	Keto Vanilla Pound Cake
15	Pork Tenderloin	Spaghetti Cottage Cheese Casserole	Garlic Chicken	Almond Roll With Pumpkin Cream Cheese Filling
16	Smoky Pork With Cabbage	Meatballs With Coconut Gravy	Lamb Shanks	No Bake Low Carb Lemon Strawberry Cheesecake
17	Italian Frittata	Fresh Dal	Jamaican Jerk Pork Roast	Pecan Cheesecake
18	Easy Mexican Chicken	Pulled Pork Salad	Salmon	Blueberry And Zucchini Muffins
19	Cherry Tomatoes Thyme	Garlic Pork Belly	Coconut Chicken	Coffee Mousse

	Asparagus Frittata			
20	Healthy Veggie Omelet	Sesame Seed Shrimp	Mahi Mahi Taco Wraps	Chocolate Cake
21	Scrambled Eggs With Smoked Salmon	Chicken Liver Pate	Shrimp Tacos	Sweet Potato Brownies
22	Persian Omelet Slow cooker	Cod Fillet In Coconut Flakes	Fish Curry	Raspberry Brownies
23	Keto Slow cooker Tasty Onions	Prawn Stew	Salmon With Creamy Lemon Sauce	Brownie Cheesecake
24	Crustless Slow cooker Spinach Quiche	Pork-Jalapeno Bowl	Salmon With Lemon-Caper Sauce	Zucchini-Brownies
25	Eggplant Pate With Breadcrumbs	Chicken Marsala	Spicy Barbecue Shrimp	Bean Brownies
26	Red Beans With The Sweet Peas	Chickpeas Soup	Lemon Dill Halibut	Luscious Walnut Chocolate Brownies
27	Nutritious Burrito Bowl	Hot And Delicious Soup	Coconut Cilantro Curry Shrimp	Gluten-Free Chocolate Cake
28	Quinoa Curry	Delicious	Shrimp In	Brownies

		Eggplant Salad	Marinara Sauce	With Nuts
29	Ham Pitta Pockets	Tasty Black Beans Soup	Garlic Shrimp	Halloween Brownies
30	Breakfast Meatloaf	Rich Sweet Potato Soup	Lemon Pepper Tilapia	Raw Brownies With Cashew Nuts

CONVERSION TABLES

Volume Equivalents (Liquid)

US STANDARD	US STANDARD (OUNCES)	METRIC (APPROXIMATE)
2 tablespoons	1 fl. oz...	30 mL
1/4 cup	2 fl. oz...	60 mL
1/2 cup	4 fl. oz...	120 mL
1 cup	8 fl. oz...	240 mL
11/2 cups	12 fl. oz...	355 mL
2 cups or 1 pint	16 fl. oz...	475 mL
4 cups or 1 quart	32 fl. oz...	1 L
1 gallon	128 fl. oz...	4 L

Volume Equivalents (Dry)

US STANDARD	METRIC (APPROXIMATE)
1/4 teaspoon	1 mL
1/2 teaspoon	2 mL
1 teaspoon	5 mL
1 tablespoon	15 mL
1/4 cup	59 mL
cup	79 mL
1/2 cup	118 mL
1 cup	177 mL

Oven Temperatures

FAHRENHEIT (F)	CELSIUS (C) (APPROXIMATE)
250°F	120 °C
300°F	150°C
325°F	165°C
350°F	180°C
375°F	190°C
400°F	200°C
425°F	220°C
450°F	230°C

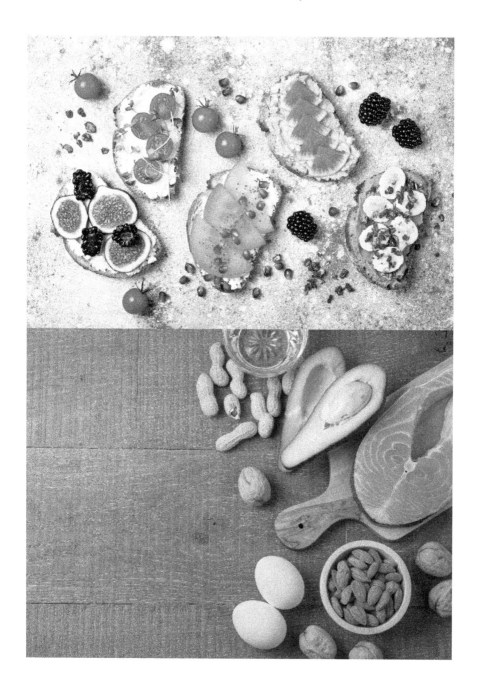

CONCLUSION

Now you can cook healthier meals for yourself, your family, and your friends that will get your metabolism running at the peak of perfection and will help you feel healthy, lose weight, and maintain a healthy balanced diet. A new diet isn't so bad when you have so many options from which to choose. You may miss your carbs, but with all these tasty recipes at your fingertips, you'll find them easily replaced with new favorites.

You will marvel at how much energy you have after sweating though the first week or so of almost no carbs. It can be a challenge, but you can do it! Pretty soon you won't miss those things that bogged down your metabolism as well as your thinking and made you tired and cranky. You will feel like you can rule the world and do anything, once your body is purged of heavy carbs and you start eating things that rejuvenate your body. It is worth the few detox symptoms when you actually start enjoying the food you are eating.

A Keto diet isn't one that you can keep going on and off. It will take your body some time to get adjusted and for ketosis to set in. This process could take anywhere between two to seven days. It is dependent on the level of activity, your body type and the food that you are eating.

There are various mobile applications that you can make use of for tracking your carbohydrate intake. There are paid and free applications as well. These apps will help you in keeping a track of your total carbohydrate and fiber intake. However, you won't be able to track your net carb intake. MyFitnessPal is one of the popular apps. You just need to open the app store on your smartphone, and you can select an app from the various apps that are available.

The amount of weight that you will lose will depend on you. If you add exercise to your daily routine, then the weight loss will be greater. If you cut down on foods that stall weight loss, then this will speed up the process. For instance, completely cutting out things like artificial sweeteners, dairy and wheat products and other related products will definitely help in speeding up your weight loss. During the first two weeks of the Keto diet, you will end up losing all the excess water weight. Ketosis has a diuretic effect on the body, and you might end up losing a couple of pounds within the first few days of this diet. After this, your body will adapt itself to burning fats for generating energy, instead of carbs.

You now have everything you need to break free from a dependence on highly processed foods, with all their dangerous additives that your body interprets as toxins. Today, when you want a sandwich for lunch, you'll roll the meat in Swiss cheese or a lettuce leaf and won't miss the bread at all, unless that is, you've made up the Keto bread recipe you discovered in this book! You can still enjoy your favorite pasta dishes, even taco salad, but without the grogginess in the afternoon that comes with all those unnecessary carbs.

So, energize your life and sustain a healthy body by applying what you've discovered. You don't have to change everything at once. Just start by adopting a new recipe each week that sounds interesting to you. Gradually, swap out less-than-healthy options for ingredients and recipes from this book that will promote your well-being.

Each time you make a healthy substitution or try a new ketogenic recipe, you can feel proud of yourself; you are actually taking good care of your mind and body. Even before you start to experience the benefits of a ketogenic lifestyle, you can feel good because you are choosing the best course for your life.

Thanks for reading.